Laser beams being used to
create a dazzling light display.

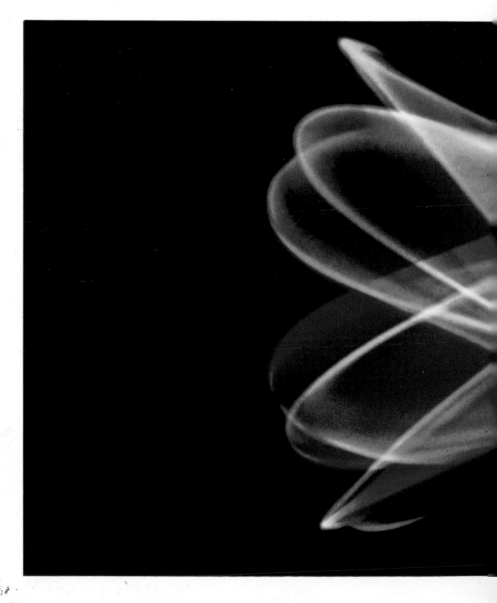

Designer	David West
Editor	James McCarter
Art Director	Charles Matheson
Typographer	Malcolm Smythe
Researcher	Dee Robinson
Consultant	Tony Search
Illustrators	Paul Cooper
	Elsa Godfrey
	Rob Shone

Designed and produced by
Aladdin Books Ltd
70 Old Compton Street
London W1

*First Published in
the United States in 1983 by*
Franklin Watts,
387 Park Avenue South,
New York, NY 10016

ISBN 0-531-04680-X

Library of Congress Catalog Card
No. 83-60900

Printed in Belgium

The Electronic Revolution

LASERS

Robin McKie

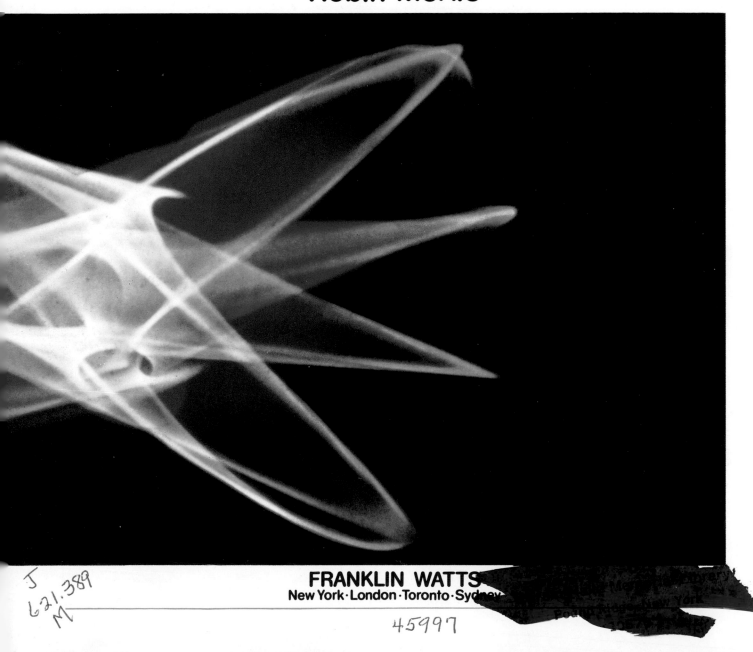

FRANKLIN WATTS
New York·London·Toronto·Sydney

Foreword

Lasers are one of the most exciting developments in 20th century science. The powerful, pencil-thin beams of light seem to belong to the world of science fiction. They conjure up pictures of death rays, living three-dimensional photographs and miraculous medical techniques.

In fact, lasers are very much part of today's world: we are already living in the laser age. Laser technology is developing rapidly and new applications are being discovered all the time. This book shows how lasers are made and explains why laser light is different from ordinary light. It shows how the unique qualities of laser light are used in science, industry, medicine, and many other walks of life.

TONY SEARCH: *Technical consultant*

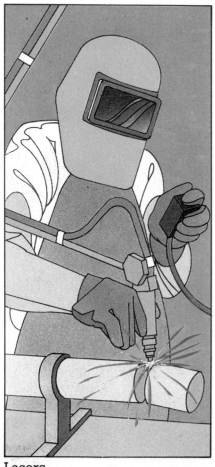

Lasers

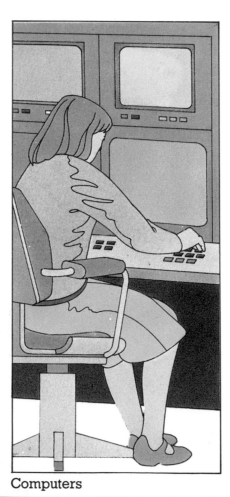

Computers

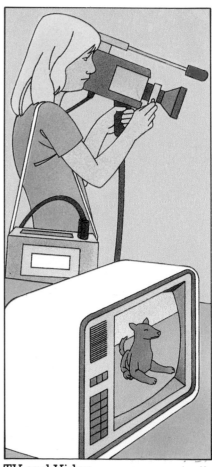

TV and Video

Contents

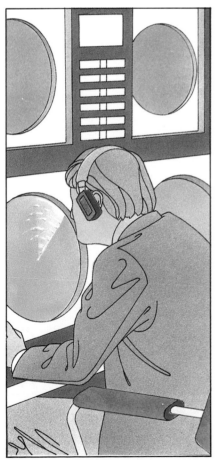

Radar and Radio

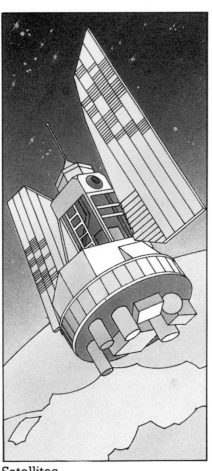

Satellites

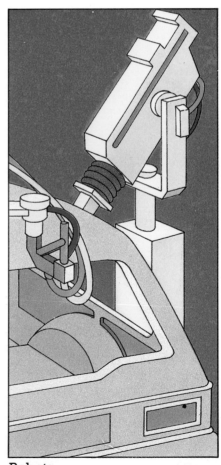

Robots

Living with lasers

The first laser was built in 1960, by scientists working in California. It contained a man-made rod of the precious crystal, ruby. When the ruby rod was subjected to very bright flashes of ordinary light, it gave out pulses of red laser light. Soon the special properties of laser light were put to use in industry, and lasers left the scientists' laboratories. Today, lasers may even be found in your local supermarket or in your own home.

Lasers in everyday life

The next time you go to the supermarket, see if the register has a laser beam to record the prices. The checkout operator will pass the goods over a laser-scanner slot or use a small laser pen. The laser "reads" a bar code printed onto a package by detecting the amount of light reflected from the background. The code, in the form of black lines, tells the computerized register the exact cost of a product. In the home, the latest video systems use laser beams to "read" video discs to create the pictures on the TV set.

▽ Bar codes (called Universal Product Codes) also contain information that helps the supermarket control its stock. The laser-scanner picks this up and sends it to a stock-control computer.

Bar code on product

0 20248 000916

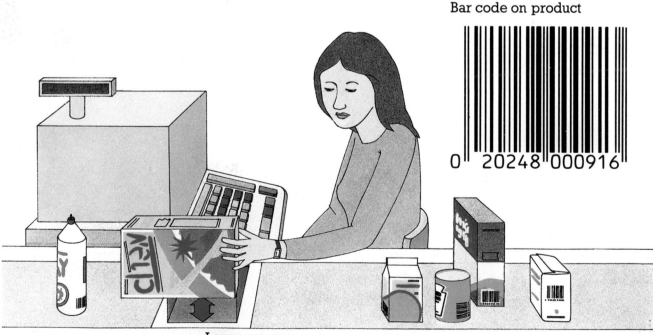

Laser-scanner

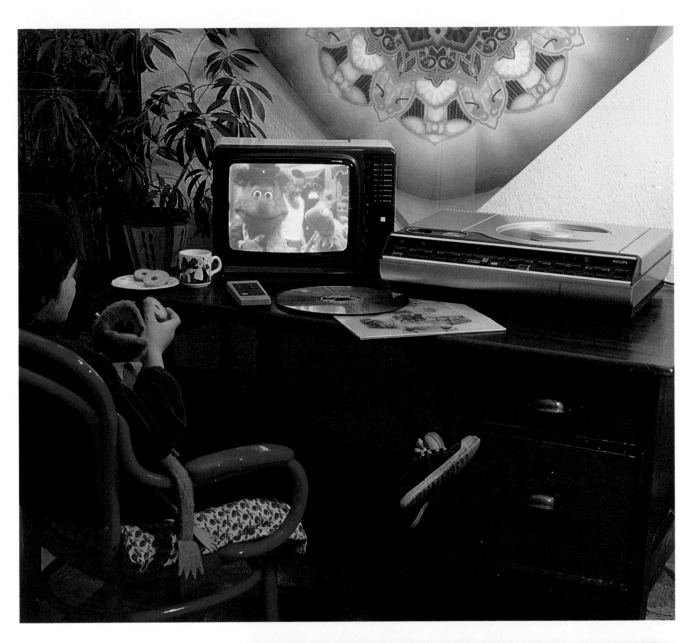

△ This video system uses a laser to read a video disc of a feature film.

▷ The laser beam detects reflections from small "pits" in the video disc. There are millions of these pits on each disc, storing all the information the video system needs to recreate TV pictures.

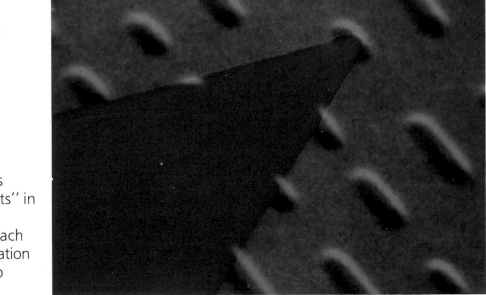

Laser light

The light we see is a form of energy that travels through the air in waves. We can't see these waves, but we can think of them as being like the waves you can make when you joggle a rope up and down. Depending on how fast you joggle the rope, you can make lots of small waves, or a few long ones. The waves of light vary in length in the same way. Long waves are those we see as red light, shorter ones are those we see as blue. The light we get from the Sun or from a flashlight is a mixture of different colors and different length light waves all jumbled together, and we see this as white light.

The waves of laser light

The waves of laser light are all one length, so lasers have one particular color. The light waves of laser light also travel beside each other, with the tops and bottoms of the waves "in step." This is what makes laser light so intense and is also the reason why laser light travels in absolutely straight, pencil-thin beams.

▽ Ordinary light contains many waves of different lengths all jumbled together. Laser light waves are all the same length and travel in step with each other. This is what gives laser light its special properties.

Light waves

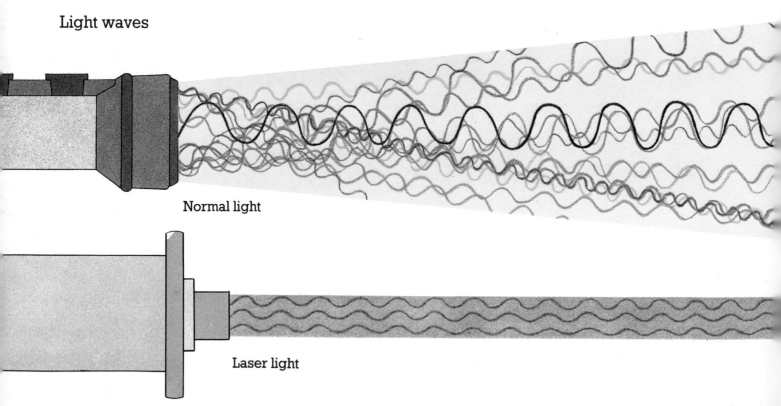

Normal light

Laser light

Splitting light

When ordinary light passes through a prism – a wedge-shaped piece of glass – it splits up into rainbow colors. This is because the light waves of different lengths – and so of different color – are bent by the prism to different degrees.

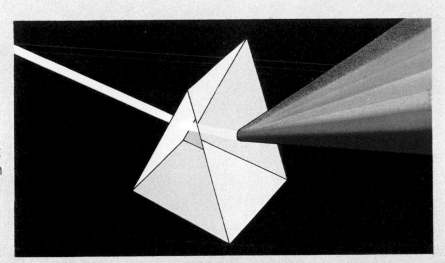

When a laser beam is passed through a prism it does not split up. If a red beam goes in, a red beam comes out. This shows that the laser light waves are all the same length and so are bent by the prism to the same degree.

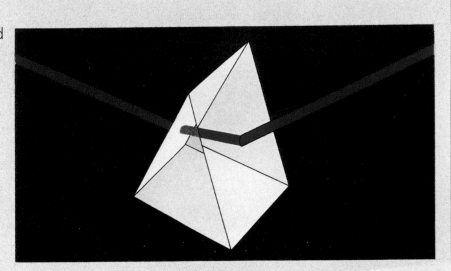

The parts of a laser

All lasers have three basic parts that make up their mechanism. First there is the *power source*. This is often electricity, but can be a strong source of ordinary light or even another laser. Next comes what is known as the *active medium*. This is the material in which the laser beam is actually generated. The active medium can be a solid material such as ruby; a liquid, such as certain dyes; or a gas such as carbon dioxide. The final part of the laser is called the *feedback mechanism*. It is made of two mirrors placed at each end of the tube in which the active medium is held. These mirrors help to amplify (build up) the intensity of the laser beam produced in the active medium.

▽ The diagram below shows a gas laser, but all other types of lasers have these basic parts.

Gas laser   Feedback mechanism

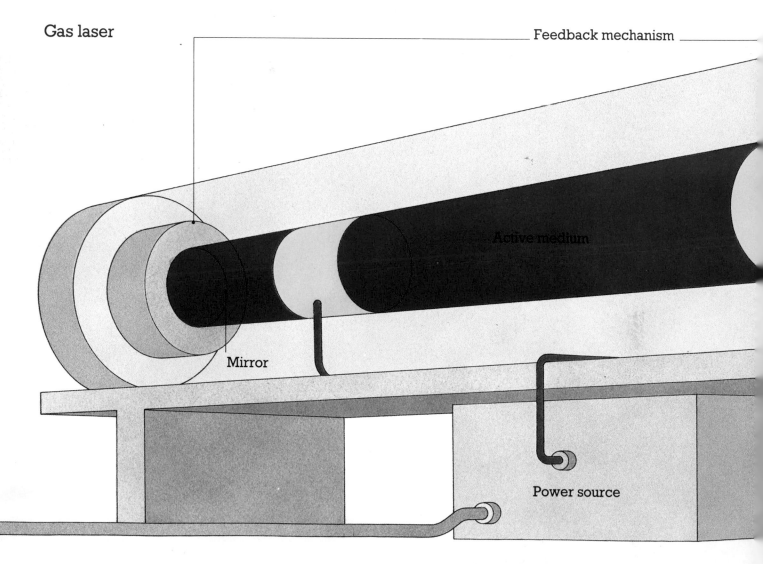

Active medium

Mirror

Power source

Different types of laser

Lasers using different active mediums produce different types of laser beams. The color of the laser beam depends on the material used. Ruby lasers produce red beams, for example, while the beam produced by a carbon dioxide laser is invisible to the naked eye. Furthermore, some lasers only give out short pulses of laser light, while others produce continuous beams. The power of the beams produced by different lasers also varies. Some can burn through sheets of metal, while others are safe enough to be used in classroom science demonstrations.

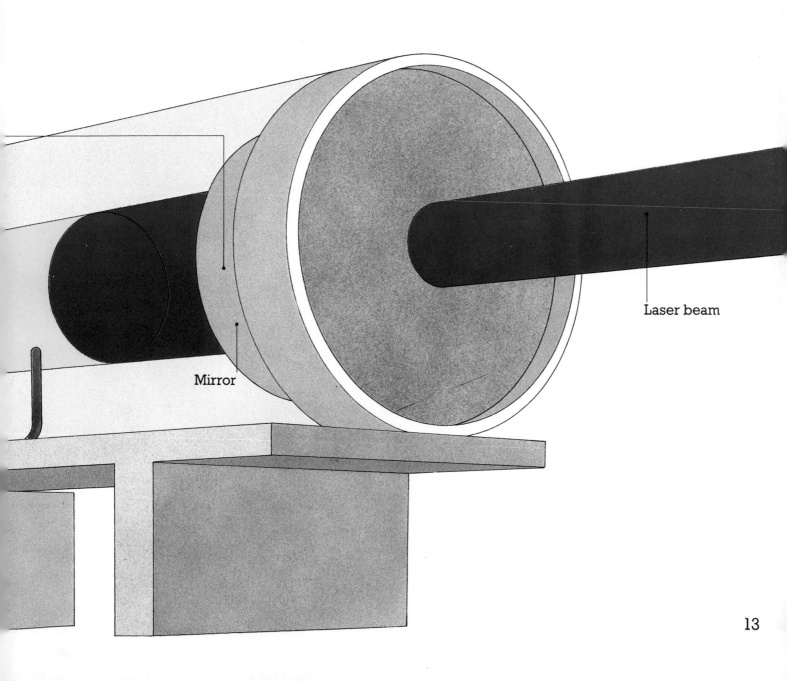

Laser beam

Mirror

Inside a laser

We've seen the parts that make up a laser, but how exactly do they work together to produce a laser beam? The answer lies within the atoms of the material used as the active medium. They absorb the energy fed into the laser by the power source. At a certain point, they have more energy than they can naturally hold. They have to get rid of this extra energy, and they do so by giving out a tiny amount of light. This part of the process is called *excitation*.

Building up the beam

Once one atom gives out light it creates a chain reaction, causing other atoms to release their energy as light. This light at first travels in all directions, but the two mirrors at each end of the laser eventually cause it to travel back and forth along the laser tube. This makes even more atoms of the active medium give out light, building up the intensity of the laser beam. The troughs and crests of each light wave coincide with all the others, so that they are almost parallel with each other. This stage of the process is called *amplification*. The output mirror at one end of the tube has a "window" in its center from which part of the laser beam can escape.

▽ The diagram below shows the three stages of creating a laser beam: (1) excitation, (2) amplification (building up the power of the beam), and (3) output of the laser.

How laser light is produced

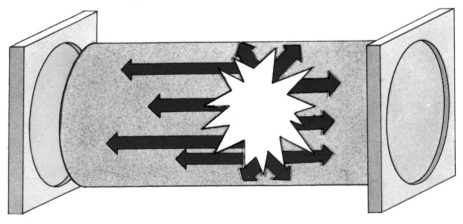

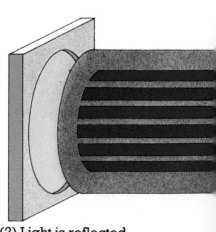

(1) First burst of light

(2) Light is reflected back and forth

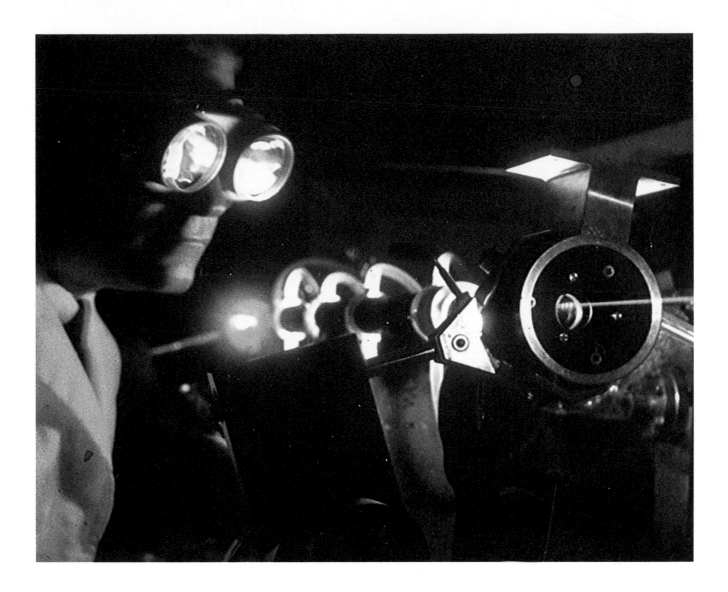

△ The laser shown here uses a
gas — argon — for its active
medium. Most gas lasers are
powered by electric currents,
although other power sources
can be used.

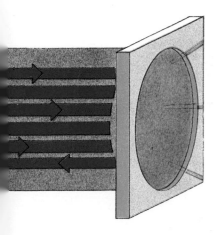

(3) Powerful light escapes as laser beam

Lasers in industry

The most powerful industrial lasers produce little more energy than the coils of an electric stove. But this energy can be focused to a point smaller than the period at the end of this sentence. Such a concentration of energy is enough to heat metals to a temperature at which they vaporize almost instantaneously. The accuracy of lasers also means that they can cut materials much more precisely than ordinary tools. And because laser light can be reflected off mirrors, it can be guided to parts that would be hard to reach by other methods.

▽ A carbon dioxide laser slices through a sheet of solid steel. Because no part of the equipment comes in touch with the metal, laser cutters do not wear out through use.

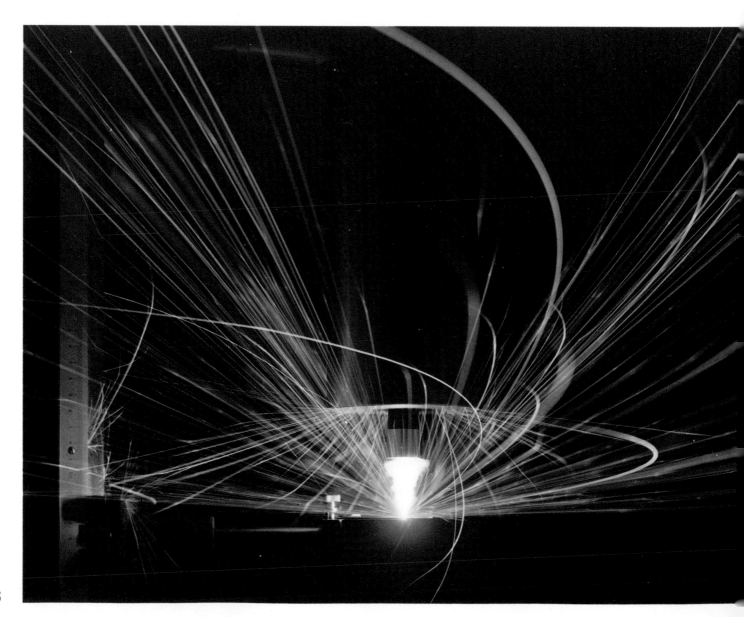

Which industries use lasers?

Lasers are used in some modern car plants – their accuracy and intensity are ideal for making the tiny "spot welds" used to assemble car bodies. But they also find their place in lighter industries, cutting paper and fabrics, or brittle substances such as glass and ceramic. And diamonds – the hardest substance known to man – can be cut with a high-power laser beam.

Building with lasers

Laser beams are perfectly straight, so engineers use them to line things up accurately. Small portable lasers are used to check that buildings are accurately constructed, to lay oil pipelines and in building bridges and tunnels.

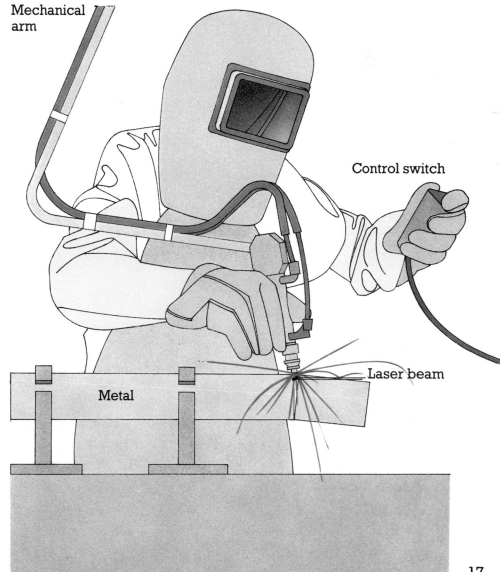

▽ Here a laser "gun" is being used to cut metal piping. The laser beam is guided by a series of mirrors in the mechanical arm. The operator's helmet protects him from sparks and the strong laser light.

Mechanical arm

Control switch

Laser beam

Metal

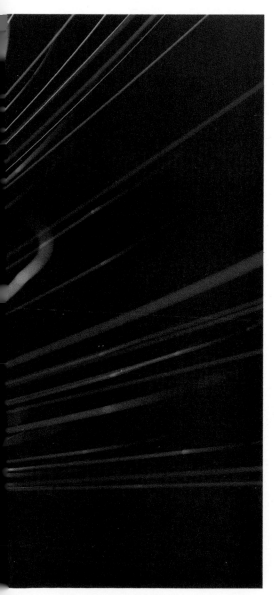

Measuring with lasers

Laser beams can be used as highly accurate measuring devices. For measuring long distances, such as the distance of the Moon from the Earth, the method is simple. Astronauts of the Apollo 11 Moon mission in 1969 left a mirror on the Moon. Pulses of laser light were aimed at it through a telescope on Earth, and the time it took for the reflected pulse to return was measured. From this, the distance of the Moon was calculated to an accuracy of 10 cm (4 inches)!

What other measurements have been made with lasers?

Laser pulses from ground stations are bounced off a satellite in fixed orbit above the Earth. From their reflection, scientists can detect and measure slight movements in the Earth's crust. But lasers don't always need mirrors or satellites to reflect them when they are used for measuring. At many international airports, lasers are bounced off clouds to measure their exact height. Lasers are used to measure very small distances as well. Scientists know the exact length of the tiny waves of laser light – usually less than a half a millionth of a metre. By counting these waves, and even small fractions of a wave, incredibly accurate measurements can be made.

▽ The San Andreas fault in California is one of the world's most populated earthquake zones. Lasers from various land stations are bounced off a satellite. Tiny movements of the Earth's crust can be measured, helping scientists to build a picture of how an earthquake happens.

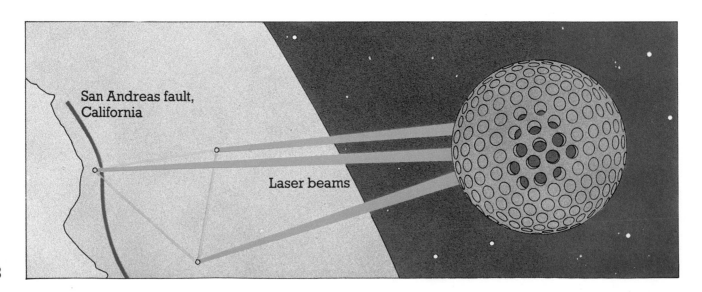

San Andreas fault, California

Laser beams

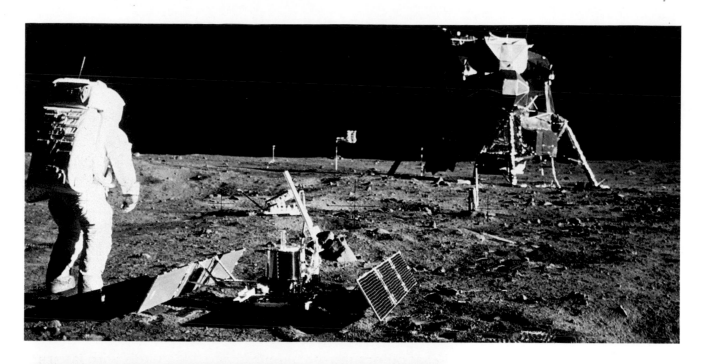

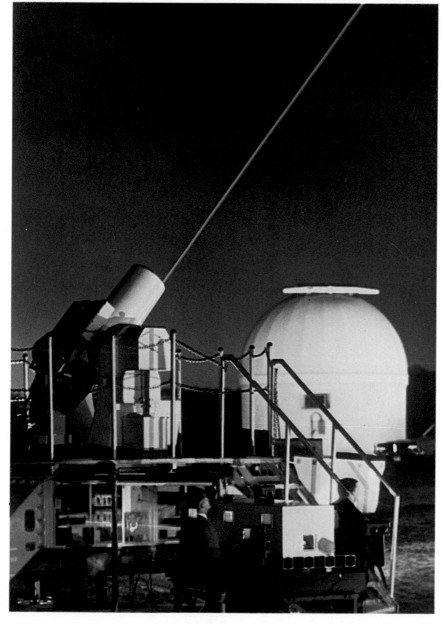

△ The mirror left by the Apollo astronauts consisted of 100 glass cubes. By the time the pencil-thin laser beam reached the Moon it had spread out to over 3 km (1.9 miles) wide. Ordinary light would have spread to thousands of kilometers, becoming too weak for a reflection to be picked up.

◁ A beam from an argon gas laser was used to measure the distance to the Moon. It was aimed at the mirror from a telescope.

Lasers in medicine

One of the first uses of lasers was in the field of medicine. Surgeons found that this new tool, which could deliver controlled amounts of energy with pin-point accuracy, was invaluable in certain delicate operations. A laser "knife" can burn away diseased tissue without damaging neighboring healthy tissue. The laser beam seals small blood vessels as it "cuts," so less blood is lost during an operation. Lasers are also completely sterile, because no part of the equipment actually touches the patient.

Eye surgery with lasers

One of the commonest uses of lasers in medicine occurs in eye surgery. At the back of our eyes is an area called the retina. The images we see fall on the retina and are carried to the brain from nerve endings there. One quite common eyesight problem is caused when the retina becomes detached from the back of the eye. Doctors can cure this with a simple laser operation. Rapid laser pulses are fired at the retina to "weld" it back into place.

▽ A surgeon uses a special laser instrument for eye surgery. The laser pulses are so rapid – about one thousand a second – that the patient does not have time to blink or move his or her head. This form of surgery is completely painless.

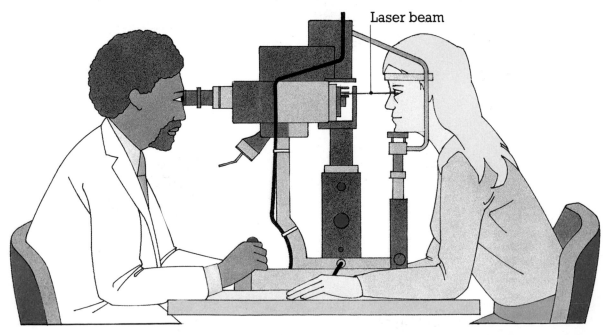

Laser beam

Doctor

Patient

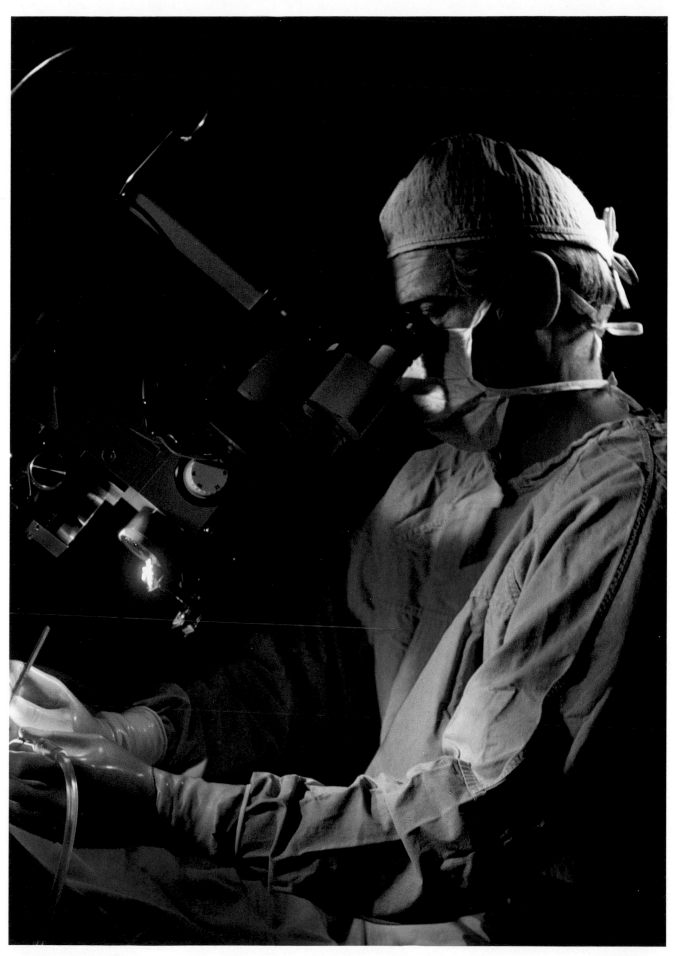

Surgeons performing ear surgery using a laser.

Lasers at war

Lasers are a vital part of the equipment of today's armed forces. Armies use laser range-finders to identify the exact position of a target – an enemy tank, for example – instantly and accurately. The range-finder works on the same principle as that used to calculate the distance to the Moon. The range-finder aims a pulse of laser light at the target. The reflected pulse is picked up and the range-finder automatically calculates the target's distance from the time the pulse took to travel. A similar but more complex system is used by some modern fighter planes to measure their altitude automatically. This enables them to fly very close to the ground to avoid detection by enemy radar.

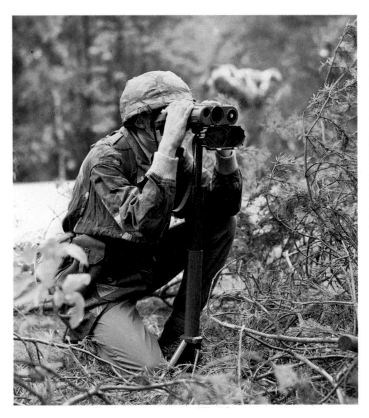

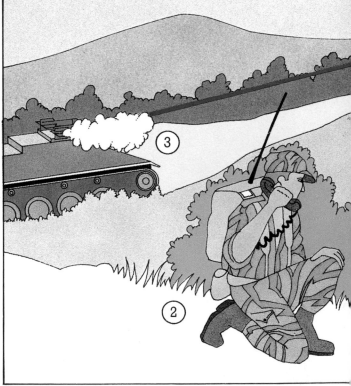

Laser range-finding
This soldier is using binocular laser range-finders. A pulse of laser light is directed at the target. The binoculars pick up the reflection and calculate the target's range.

"Spotlighting" a target by laser

Lasers are also used to guide missiles to their targets. Soldiers on the ground use a device called a "laser target designator" to spotlight the target. This sends out tiny, invisible laser pulses which bounce off the target in all directions. The reflected pulses are picked up by a special receiver in the nose cone of the missile, which uses them to home in on the target.

Can lasers be used as weapons themselves?

People often think of lasers as "death ray" weapons, similar to those seen in films such as *Star Wars*. In fact, laser technology has a long way to go before these weapons become reality. Laser beams travel at the speed of light – 300,000 kilometers per second (186,000 miles per second) – and might be able to knock out enemy missiles as soon as they were launched.

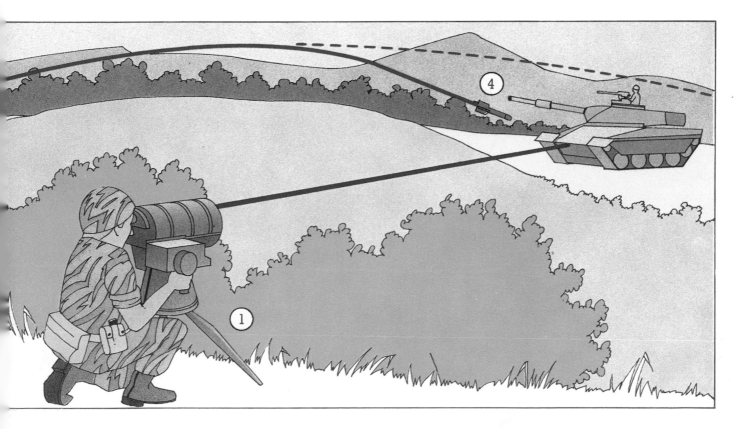

Laser target designation
Soldiers aim the laser designator (1) at an enemy tank. The laser is invisible to the enemy soldiers.

When the target has been engaged by the laser, the commander radios his artillery unit (2). The laser-guided missile is then launched (3).

The missile uses the reflected laser beam to find its target (4). The missile's normal flight path is shown by the dotted line.

Laser art

The brilliant colors of laser beams have been used in displays all over the world. Rock groups often include a laser light show as part of their performance. The laser beams used in public displays are not powerful, and precautions are taken to make sure that they cannot shine into people's eyes.

Laser photography – Holograms

Holograms are a special type of photograph that can only be made using lasers. Holograms record three-dimensional images that look just like solid objects when viewed. When you look at a hologram, the image changes as you change your position of viewing, just as it does when you look at objects in real life.

How are holograms made?

Holograms are created by illuminating objects with laser light. They are recorded on either film or glass plates. To view the hologram, a laser beam, or in some cases ordinary white light, is shone on the film or plate to reveal the image.

▷ Many museums run permanent laser light shows. The intensity of the laser beam can produce dramatic and beautiful displays.

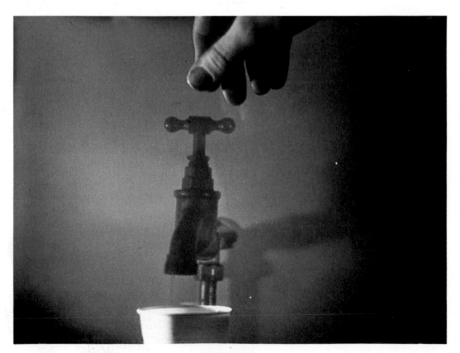

◁ Holograms seem to be as real as solid objects – until you reach out to try and touch them. In this photograph the hand and cup are real, but the tap is a hologram image.

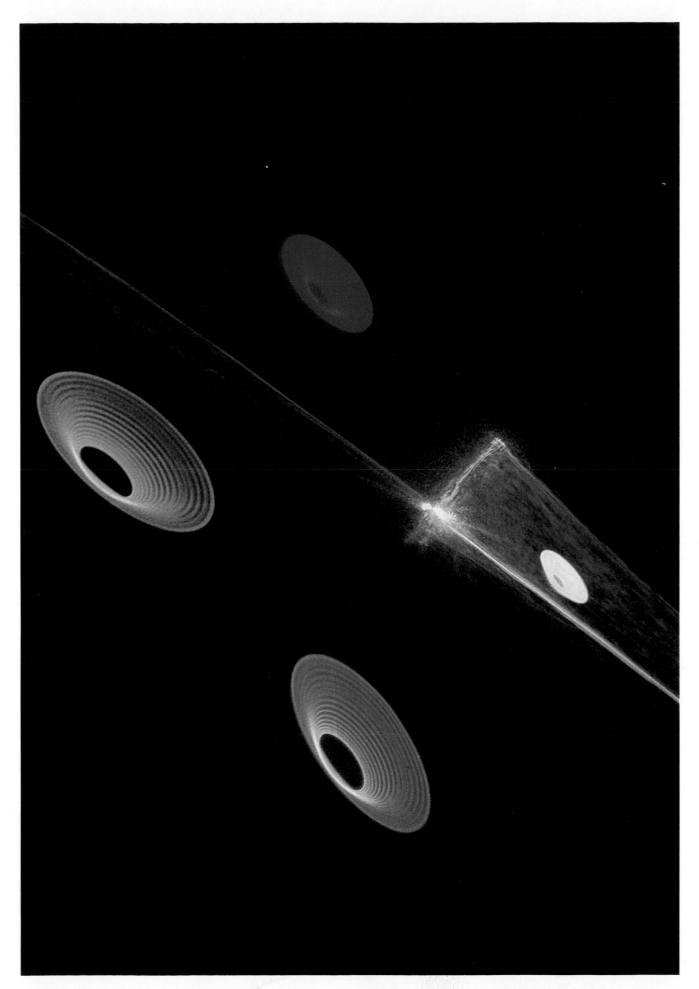

Laser developments

In the future, lasers could become almost as important to our everyday lives as electricity is at present. Tiny flexible cables, called "fiber optics," can transmit laser light over great distances. The light reflects off the inner walls of the fiber and can be used to carry information. A telephone network of optical fibers for example, can carry many more calls than one using ordinary electrical telephone cables. Such networks are already being installed.

A new source of power

Scientists are experimenting with lasers to create a new source of power. When the gas hydrogen is heated to temperatures of many millions of degrees, it changes into another element called helium and releases even more heat. It is this process – known as *fusion* – which powers the Sun. By using highly powerful lasers, scientists hope to create miniature "suns" on Earth, giving us an almost limitless supply of energy. One experiment uses 20 lasers firing at the same time to achieve the temperatures necessary for fusion.

▽ In an optical fiber telephone network, voices are converted into electrical signals, and then into tiny pulses of laser light. Devices known as "repeaters" boost the laser signal to enable it to travel great distances. At the receiving end, the signal is converted back into speech.

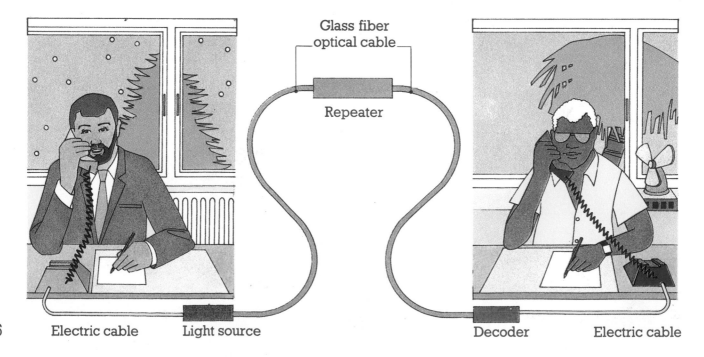

Glass fiber optical cable

Repeater

Electric cable   Light source   Decoder   Electric cable

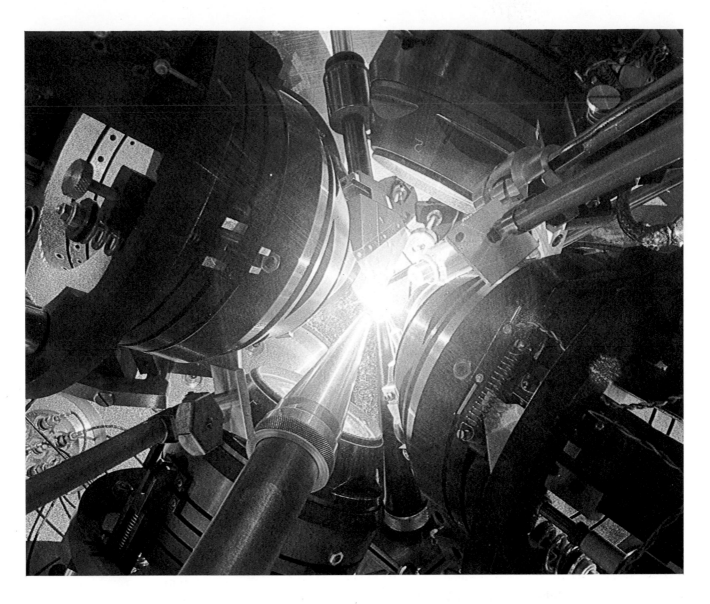

△ Laser fusion in action at the Rutherford laboratory in Cambridge, England.

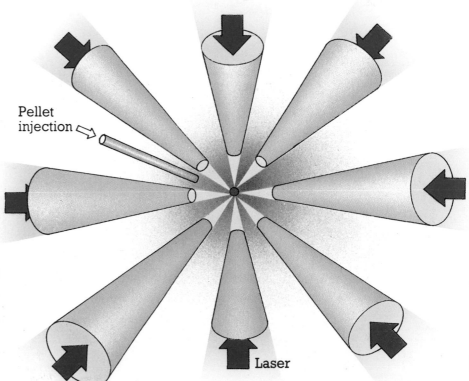

Pellet injection ⇨

Laser

▷ High-power laser beams are focused on a small pellet of frozen hydrogen. The pellet is heated to millions of degrees almost instantly and fusion takes place.

Glossary

Active medium The part of the laser which generates light when energy is put in from the power source.

Atom A tiny particle of matter from which solids, liquids and gases are made. Many millions of atoms make up the period at the end of this sentence.

Carbon dioxide A gas which is part of the air that we breathe and which can be used as an active medium in lasers.

Excitation The process by which atoms absorb energy and then give it out as light.

Feedback mechanisms The name for the two mirrors at either end of a laser. Light is bounced between these two mirrors until it is released as a laser beam.

Fiber-optics Very thin glass rods through which pulses of light can be sent.

Hologram A three dimensional picture made by shining lasers on an object and recording the reflections on a plate or film.

Laser A machine that emits powerful beams of light. The name is short for Light Amplification by Stimulated Emission of Radiation – the proper scientific name for a laser.

Laser target designator A device used by soldiers to mark enemy targets by shining lasers on them. Laser-guided missiles can then be fired at them.

Prism A wedge-shaped piece of glass which splits up white light into different colors.

Pulse A fleeting signal that might last only a millionth of a second.

Index

Acknowledgments

The publishers wish to thank the following people who have helped in the preparation of this book:
Barr & Stroud, Bell Laboratories, Coherent, Eve Richer/Quicksilver, Ferranti, Good Relations Group, Hughes Aircraft Corp, Lasergage Ltd, Light Fantastic, Marconi, NCR Ltd, Philips, Rockwell International, Spectra-Physics.

Photographic Credits:

Cover: Coherent UK, *title page*: Bill Reber, page 9: David West; Paul Brierley, page 15: Photri, page 17: Hughes Aircraft Company, page 19: NASA; Photri, page 21: Spectra-Physics, page 22 Lasergage, page 24: Theo Bergstrom; Laser Images, page 27: Rutherford-Appleton Laboratory.